国際学会 English

ポケット版

Key sentences for presentations

C. S. Langham（日本大学特任教授）著

医歯薬出版株式会社

This book is originally published in Japanese under the title of :

KOKUSAI GAKKAI ENGLISH POCKET-BAN
(Key Sentences for Presentations)

C. S. Langham
Professor at Nihon University

ISHIYAKU PUBLISHERS, INC.
7-10, Honkomagome 1 chome, Bunkyo-ku,
Tokyo 113-8612, Japan

Introduction

This book provides a handy list of key sentences for oral presentations, poster presentations, the question and answer session, chairperson English, and acting as a master of ceremonies at a banquet. It is designed so that readers can get quick and easy access to key sentences that will be of use at international conferences. The sentences in this book are linked to the 国際学会 English series, which offers more detailed information and further examples of the situations covered here.

The material in this book has been developed over a period of 25 years, and I am extremely grateful for the invitations to speak at conferences, and the feedback that it has generated. I hope that you will find it useful.

Clive Langham

Nihon University,
School of Dentistry,
Ochanomizu, Tokyo
July 1 st, 2022

本書掲載例文の出典

本書は，「国際学会 English　挨拶・口演・発表・質問・座長進行」，「国際学会 English　ポスター発表」，「国際学会 English　口頭発表　研究発表のための英語プレゼンテーション」に掲載されている例文を抜粋・再編成したものです．各例文の下には参照ページを記載していますので，詳しい解説や関連する他の例文については，各書籍をご参照ください．

国際学会 English
挨拶・口演・発表・質問・座長進行

C.S. Langham 著
B6 判 /210 頁 /2 色刷
2007 年 4 月発行
ISBN 978-4-263-43333-1

●口演（口頭発表），ポスター発表，質疑応答，座長進行，懇親会の司会，グループディスカッションなど，国際学会のさまざまな場面で使われる英語表現を網羅しています．例文とその解説だけではなく，プレゼンテーションのテクニック向上のためのアドバイスも多数掲載しています．

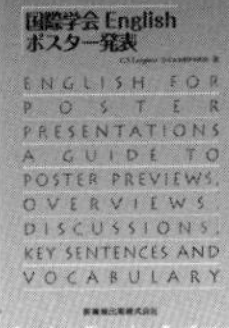

国際学会 English
ポスター発表

C.S. Langham 著
A5 判 /128 頁 /2 色刷
2013 年 8 月発行
ISBN 978-4-263-43354-6

●ポスター発表に特化した 1 冊です．ポスタープレビューにおける発表内容紹介，ポスターの概要の説明，聴衆との質疑応答や討論，受賞スピーチなどで使われる英語表現と，分かりやすいポスター発表を行うためのポイントを紹介しています．

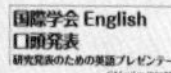

国際学会 English　口頭発表
研究発表のための英語プレゼンテーション

C.S. Langham 著
A5 判 /240 頁 /2 色刷
2019 年 12 月発行
ISBN 978-4-263-43364-5

●口頭発表の始め方と終わり方，文章量が多すぎるスライドをすっきりとまとめ直す方法，書き言葉の英語を話し言葉の英語に変換する方法，日本人が間違いやすい英文法など，一段上のプレゼンテーションを目指すために押さえておきたいポイントが満載です．

その他の関連書籍

国際学会 English スピーキング・エクササイズ
口演・発表・応答 音声 CD 付

C.S. Langham 著
A5 判 / 120 頁 / 2 色刷
2010 年 3 月発行
ISBN 978-4-263-43339-3

国際論文 English　査読・執筆ハンドブック

C.S. Langham 著
A5 判 / 160 頁 / 2 色刷
2011 年 10 月発行
ISBN 978-4-263-43347-8

国際論文 English　投稿ハンドブック
カバーレター作成・査読コメントへの返答

C.S. Langham 著
A5 判 / 184 頁 / 2 色刷
2017 年 1 月発行
ISBN 978-4-263-43361-4

目次

I 口頭発表

■ 発表の始め方

「ご紹介ありがとうございます.」

- Thank you.
- Thank you, chair.
- Thank you, chairperson.
- Thank you, Professor Williams.
- Thank you for your introduction.
- Thank you very much for your kind introduction.

● はじめに座長へのお礼を述べる. 上記のとおりさまざまな言い方があるが, 学会発表においては短い表現が好まれるため, 手短に Thank you と言うのが最も望ましい.

▷挨拶・口演・発表・質問・座長進行, p.6
▷口頭発表, p.2, 21, 28

『（招待講演などの場合）本日は，このような機会をいただき大変光栄に思います．』

- **It is a great honor to be able to speak to you today.**
- **It gives me great pleasure to speak to you today.**
- **I'm very happy to be able to talk to you today.**
- **I'm very pleased to have this opportunity to speak to you today.**

● 招待講演などの場合，講演を始める前に，opening comments として上記のように述べる．

● 講演の規模や公式な場であるかどうかに応じて表現を使い分ける．1番目の例文が最も改まった表現である．

▷挨拶・口演・発表・質問・座長進行，p.7

「(招待講演などの場合) 本日講演の機会をいただけたことに感謝申し上げます.」

- I would like to express my thanks to (name/organization) for inviting me to speak here today.
- Before I start, I would like to thank (name/organization) for inviting me to speak today. It's a pleasure to be here.
- I'd like to thank (name/organization) for kindly inviting me to speak here today.
- Before I start, I'd like to say a big thank you to the organizers for inviting me.
- I'd like to say that it is a great pleasure and an honor to be invited to speak here today.
- Thank you very much for giving me the opportunity to speak at this conference.

● 招待講演などの場合，大会長や実行委員会に対し，講演の場を設けてくれたことに対するお礼を述べる．

▷挨拶・口演・発表・質問・座長進行，p.8
▷口頭発表，p.50

「～大学の～と申します.」

- My name is Ken Watanabe. I'm with London University. I'm in the Department of Informatics.
- I'm Ken Williams. I'm with the University of Wales. I'm in the Department of Operative Dentistry.
- I'm Ken Wilson. I'm with King's College, London in the Department of Community Health.
- I'm Ken Wilson. I work at Kings College, London in the Department of Community Health.

● 自己紹介として，名前と所属を述べる.

● 所属する大学や研究機関はI'm withやI work at，学部名や部門名はI'm inで紹介する．3番目，4番目の例文のように，両者をまとめて1文で述べることもできる.

▷口頭発表，p.3, 11, 37

「私達は～（大まかな研究領域）の研究を行っています．」

- We have been working on ways of helping people at high risk of diabetes.
- We have been doing research on (topic).
- We have been focusing on (topic).

● 自己紹介における研究内容の紹介は，大まかな研究領域→具体的な研究テーマ，の順番で行う．

▷口頭発表，p.32

「私達は特に，～（具体的な研究テーマ）について研究しています．」

- Our main focus is community projects where pre-diabetic people meet with health workers in the community.
- We are working on (topic).
- We are particularly interested in (topic).

● 大まかな研究領域を述べた後，より具体的な内容を説明する．

▷口頭発表，p.33

「本日は～についてお話しします.」

- Today, I'm going to talk about the role of iron plaque.
- Today, I'd like to talk about (topic).
- Today, I want to talk about (topic).
- Today, I will focus on (topic).
- In this presentation, I'd like to focus on (topic).
- My presentation today is about (topic).
- My presentation today is on (topic).

● 自己紹介に続いて発表テーマを紹介する．この際，正式な発表タイトル全文を読み上げる必要はない．タイトルから重要なキーワードをいくつか抜き出して手短に紹介するとよい．

▷挨拶・口演・発表・質問・座長進行，p.11
▷口頭発表，p.6, 21

『（目次スライドを提示して）**こちらが本日の発表の目次です．**』

- **This is an outline.**
- **Here are the contents.**
- **These are the contents.**
- **Here are the points I'm going to cover.**
- **These are the topics I'm going to cover.**
- **Today, I'll be covering these points/topics.**
- **Today, I'm going to cover these topics.**
- **These are the main points I'll cover today.**

● 目次スライドがある場合は，目次に沿って発表の概略を紹介する．はじめに目次の紹介を始める合図として上記のように言う．

▷口頭発表，p.12, 28

「本日は～つのパートに分けてお話ししたいと思います.」

- As you can see, my presentation has 5 parts.
- My presentation is in 5 parts.
- This presentation is divided into 5 parts.
- Today, I will be looking at 5 parts.

● 発表全体がいくつのパートに分かれるかを最初に示すことで，聴衆が全体の構成を把握しやすくなる.

▷挨拶・口演・発表・質問・座長進行，p.12
▷口頭発表，p.22

「はじめに～についてお話しします.」

- I'll start by focusing on forms of radiocesium released from FDNPs.
- I'll start with an introduction to (topic).
- First, I'll look at (topic).
- I'll begin by looking at (topic).
- In part 1, I'll talk about (topic).

● 目次スライドの紹介では，各パートの概略を順番に説明していく.

▷口頭発表，p.13, 29

「まず／次に／それから／最後に，～についてお話しします．」

- First/Firstly, I'm going to talk about (topic).
- Second/Secondly, I want to consider/explain (topic).
- Then, I'd like to focus on (topic).
- Lastly/Finally, I'll review the main findings of this study.

● 各パートの概略を順に説明していく際は，上記のように順序を表す表現を活用するとよい．

▷挨拶・口演・発表・質問・座長進行，p.13

「続いて，～についてお話しします．」

- I'll move on to interventions for pre-diabetics.
- I'll go on to interventions for pre-diabetics.
- Next, I'll look at interventions for pre-diabetics.

● 「次の話題に移る」と言いたい時は，move on to や go on to を使うとよい．

▷口頭発表，p.14

『～についてもお話しします．』

- I will also look at distribution and speciation of Cd around iron plaque.
- I will also discuss (topic).
- I will also consider (topic)

● 「さらに～についても」と言いたい時は also を使用する．

▷口頭発表，p.24

『それでは，はじめにこの研究の背景を説明します．』

- I'd like to start with some background.
- Let's look at some background.
- I'll just run through some background.
- I'd like to mention the background of/to this study.
- I'll start by explaining some background.

● 目次スライドの紹介を終え，研究背景の説明に移るときは，上記のように言う．

▷口頭発表，p.41，43

「～についてはこれまで多くの研究が行われてきました.」

- There has been a lot of work on improving memory or slowing down memory loss in old people.
- Most studies have focused on light exercise as a way of reducing risk of dementia.
- A lot of research has focused on (topic).
- There are several studies on (topic).
- The majority of studies have looked at (topic).

● 研究の背景・目的の説明にあたっては,「先行研究によって○○が明らかになっている」→「しかし△△についてはまだよく分かっていない」→「そこで△△を明らかにするため,本研究を行った」という流れで説明するのが一般的である.はじめに,これまでどのような先行研究が行われてきたのかを説明する.

▷口頭発表, p.44, 45

「現在，～ということが明らかになっています．」
「～ということはよく知られています．」

- **Currently, we know that** light exercise is a good way of preventing memory loss.
- **A lot of studies have reported that** the number of people who want to improve the appearance of their teeth is increasing.
- **It is well known that** the number of people who want to improve the appearance of their teeth is increasing.

● 先行研究の結果どのようなことが明らかになったのかを簡単に紹介する．

▷口頭発表，p.38, 46

「しかし，～についてはまだ分かっていません.」

- But we don't know much about levels of post-treatment patient satisfaction.
- However, there are only a few studies on levels of post-treatment patient satisfaction.
- But, there is not much in the literature on levels of post-treatment patient satisfaction.
- No studies have focused on the benefits of light exercise on memory.
- There has been no work on the benefits of light exercise on memory.
- Studies on the benefits of light exercise on memory have been limited to slow walking.

● 先行研究の紹介に続いて，「まだ分かっていないこと」を紹介する．この「まだ分かっていないこと」は，research gap（研究ギャップ）や research niche（研究ニッチ）とよばれる．

▷口頭発表，p.39, 47

「この研究の目的は，〜です．」

- We wanted to see how patients evaluated the products they used.
- Our objective was to find out how patients reacted to different products.
- The main aim was to investigate nitrates in rivers.
- One of the main goals of this study was to assess the potential benefits of light exercise.
- The main motivation of this study was to assess the potential benefits of light exercise.
- The objective of this study was to assess the potential benefits of light exercise.

●研究の目的は上記のように紹介する．

▷口頭発表，p.40, 47

「～について調べました.」

- We looked at three commercial whitening products.
- We focused on three commercial whitening products.
- We investigated three commercial whitening products.
- We studied levels of patient satisfaction.
- We concentrated on levels of patient satisfaction.

● 「調べる／研究する」を表す動詞としては，口頭発表では look at や focus on などの句動詞を用いることが多い.

▷口頭発表，p.40

「それでは，はじめに〜についてお話しします．」

- I'd like to start by talking about (topic).
- I want to begin by discussing (topic).
- I'll start by giving an overview of (topic).
- I'll start by focusing on (topic).
- I'm going to start by talking about (topic).
- I'll start by looking at (topic).

● 自己紹介や目次の紹介を終えた後，発表の本題に入る時は上記のように言う．

▷挨拶・口演・発表・質問・座長進行，p.14
▷口頭発表，p.25, 52

発表で使える便利な表現

「このセクションでは，～についてお話ししたいと思います．」

- In this section, I'm going to talk about/discuss/consider/examine (topic).
- In this part of my presentation, I'd like to tell you about (topic).
- Now, I'm going to give an overview of (topic).

● 各セクションの冒頭では，このセクションで話す内容を簡単に述べると，聴衆が発表の流れを把握しやすくなる．

▷挨拶・口演・発表・質問・座長進行，p.24

「このスライドは，～について示しています．」

- Here, we have (data/information).
- Here, you can see (data/information).
- This slide shows (data/information).

● スライドが替わったら，まず Here を使ってそのスライドの概要を示すとよい．

▷挨拶・口演・発表・質問・座長進行，p.41

『このスライドのポイントは，～ということです．』

- The key point here is that the substrate is thinner and more flexible.
- The key issue here is that the substrate is thinner and more flexible.
- So, the main point in this slide is that the substrate is thinner and more flexible.
- The main message here is that the substrate is thinner and more flexible.
- The take-home message from this data is that the substrate is thinner and more flexible.

● 各スライドの説明の最後に，そのスライドの要点を簡単に振り返ると聴衆の理解が深まる．

▷口頭発表，p.170

「ここでいったん，ここまでの数枚のスライドのまとめをいたします．ポイントは～です．」

- We have covered quite a lot of ground. So I'd like to summarize what we have seen in the last few slides. (short summary of the main points)
- I'd like to summarize what we have seen in the last few slides. The main points are (short summary of the main points).
- This is what we have seen in the last few slides. (short summary of the main points)

● スライド１枚１枚についてではなく，スライド数枚分のまとめを述べてもよい．

▷口頭発表，p.170

『このセクションのまとめをいたします．ポイントは～です．』

- I'd like to wrap up this section by summarizing the main points. (review of 2~3 points)
- I'd like to summarize the main points of this section. (review of 2~3 points).
- I'll just go over the main points in this section. (review of 2~3 points)
- The main points of this section are these. (review of 2~3 points).
- The key points here are as follows. (review of 2~3 points).

● 各セクションの終わりに要点をまとめると，聴衆もより理解が増す．

● 句動詞 wrap up は「要約する，まとめる」などの意味をもち，学会発表でまとめを述べる際に便利な表現である．

▷挨拶・口演・発表・質問・座長進行，p.27
▷口頭発表，p.171

「続いて，～についてお話しします．」

- **Next, I'm going to move on to** the results and discussion.
- **Now, I'm going to go on to** the results and discussion.
- **Next, I'm going to look at** the results and discussion.
- **Next, I'd like to move on to** results and discussion.
- **Next, I want to go on to** (topic).
- **Now, I will move on to the next section and talk about** (topic).

● 新しい話題に移る時は，そのことを聴衆に示す必要がある．次の話題に移ることを示す表現として，move on to や go on to などの句動詞が便利である．

▷口頭発表，p.102
▷挨拶・口演・発表・質問・座長進行，p.29

「～については次のスライドでご説明します.」

- I'll show you the approaches we used in the next slide.
- I'll focus on that data in the next slide.
- In the next slide, I'll summarize data from our experiments.
- So, the main issue is reliability. I'll talk about that in the next slide.
- So, the main issue is reliability. I'll focus on that in the next slide.

● 次のスライドで話す内容を予告することで，聴衆が発表の流れを把握しやすくなる.

▷口頭発表，p.103, 136
▷挨拶・口演・発表・質問・座長進行，p.40

「次の数枚のスライドでは，～についてご説明します．」

- In the next few slides, I want to focus on reliability.
- In the next three slides, I'll discuss the issue of reliability.
- I'll show you some data on reliability in the next few slides.
- Over the next few slides, I'll focus on reliability.

● 続く数枚のスライドの内容が共通している場合は，上記のようにまとめて紹介してもよい．

▷口頭発表，p.105

『～については後ほど／次のセクションでお話しします．』

- **I'll return to this issue later.**
- **I'll talk about the significance of this result in the next section.**
- **I'll give you more information about that in the next section.**
- **I'm going to give you more details about that in the next section.**
- **I'll come back to this point in the discussion.**

● 「後ほど」「次のセクションで」「考察のセクションで」などのように，後で話す内容を予告する場合は上記のように言う．

▷口頭発表，p.137
▷挨拶・口演・発表・質問・座長進行，p.30

「これで～についての話しは終わりです.」

- That's all I have to say about (topic).
- That covers what I want to say about (topic).
- That concludes this section.

● 各セクションの終わりをはっきり示すことで，聴衆が発表の流れを把握しやすくなる.

▷挨拶・口演・発表・質問・座長進行，p.28

「一方，～（今まで説明していたのとは別の話題）については，～です.」

- In terms of energy consumption, it is marginally more efficient.
- As far as energy consumption is concerned, it is marginally more efficient.
- From the viewpoint of energy consumption, it is marginally more efficient.

● 「一方，～については」という形で新しい話題に移るときは，In terms of や As far as を使うのが簡単である.

▷口頭発表，p.110

『先ほど～のところでお話ししたとおり，～です.』

- As I mentioned in the background, typical lifespans for this product are between 5 to 7 years.
- As I explained in the introduction, (repetition of fact/data).
- As I pointed out at the beginning of my talk, (repetition of fact/data).
- As we saw previously, (repetition of fact/data).

『～についてお話しした内容をもう一度振り返りたいと思います.』

- I'd like to go back to what I said about medical applications.
- I'm going to go back to the experimental setup and remind you of the major differences between these systems.

● 一度話した内容を繰り返すことで，現在の話題との関連が明確になる.

▷口頭発表，p.138, 140
▷挨拶・口演・発表・質問・座長進行，p.31

「（レーザーポインターで指しながら）これは～を示しています．」

- **Here we have** the main results.
- **Here we have** the experimental setup.
- **Here is** the experimental setup.

● レーザーポインターで指した箇所について「これは～」と説明する時は上記のように言う．

▷口頭発表，p.107

「～にご注目ください．この図表／データから～であることが分かります．」

- **Let's take a look at** the experimental setup. **As you have probably noticed,** there is a reduction in size.
- **Let's look at** the bar chart. **As you have probably seen,** rates are fairly consistent.
- **Please look at** the precipitation data. **As you have probably noted,** June has become progressively drier.

● スライド内の注目箇所を示すには，上記のように言う．レーザーポインターで該当箇所を指しながら言うとよい．

▷口頭発表，p.144

『～にご注目ください．これは～を示しています．』

- One thing to note is the sudden decrease at this point. This indicates a change in the structure of the material.
- Please note the sudden decrease at this point. This indicates a change in the structure of the material.
- As you have probably noted, there is a sudden decrease at this point. This indicates that the molecules are in an excited state.
- I guess that many of you will have already noted that there is a sudden decrease at this point. This shows that the molecules are in an excited state.

● 上記の例文はいずれも，1文目で図表内の注目箇所を示し，2文目でそれが何を示しているかを説明している．

▷口頭発表，p.147

「～をご覧いただくと，～であることが分かります.」

- If you look at this red line, you will see that degradation increases rapidly after day 3.
- If you look at this data, you will notice that degradation increases rapidly after day 3.
- If you look at the results for experiment 3, you will see a sudden increase in dopamine.

● スライド内のどこに注目してほしいかを示す時，この例のようにIfを使うこともできる.

▷口頭発表，p.145

「～という結果を得ました.」

- With the modified device, using magnesium alloys, **we achieved** a significant reduction in power consumption.
- **We obtained** a significant reduction in power consumption.
- **We got** a significant reduction in power consumption.
- **There was** a significant reduction in power consumption.

● 「結果を得た」を表す動詞は achieved や obtained が一般的であるが，学会発表においてはややくだけた表現として got も使用できる．

▷口頭発表，p.153

「また，～という結果も得られました.」

- At the same time, we saw an increase in efficiency.
- We also observed an increase in efficiency.
- There were also increases in quality, reliability, and strength.
- Another thing we noted was an increase in reliability.
- We also noted increases in quality, reliability and strength.

● 追加で結果を述べる際は，At the same time（同時に）や Also，In addition を用いる.

▷口頭発表，p.153, 154, 155

『～のデータは含まれておりません.』

- That is the data from experiments 1 and 2. We actually did one other experiment, but that data is not included here.
- I did not include that data.
- That data is not shown.
- There were some other results that I have not included here.

●結果を示す図表に一部のデータが含まれていないこともある．その場合は上記のように説明する．

▷口頭発表，p.156

「この結果から〜ということが読み取れます.」

- As you can see from the data I have presented, there is an increase in temperature and reaction speed.
- What we have seen from this data is that there is an increase in temperature and reaction speed.

● 結果を示す図表から何が読み取れるか（例：数値の上昇）を説明する際は，上記のような表現を用いる.

▷口頭発表，p.172

「この結果は，〜ということを意味しています.」

- This means that molecules are excited and move freely.
- This suggests that molecules are excited and move freely.
- So, these results tell us that molecules are excited and move freely.

● グラフや数値をもとに実験結果／調査結果を説明した後は，その結果がどのような意味をもっているかを説明する.

▷口頭発表，p.173

「この結果は何を意味しているのでしょうか？」

- **What do the results mean?**
- **What do these figures mean?**
- **What does the sudden increase in temperature mean?**
- **How can we interpret this data?**
- **What do these results tell us about the mechanism?**
- **What is the significance of these results?**
- **What do these figures tell us about productivity?**
- **What can we conclude from this figure / chart?**

●学会発表においては，疑問形をうまく活用することで聴衆の興味を引きつけることができる．

▷口頭発表，p.116, 151
▷挨拶・口演・発表・質問・座長進行，p.45

「〜の原因ははっきりしません.」

- We (still) don't know why the reaction was unsuccessful.
- We are not sure why the reaction was unsuccessful.
- We don't know the reason for the sudden increase in temperature.

● 結果の考察においては，なぜそのような結果が得られたのかを説明することが必要である．原因を説明できない場合には，上記のように述べる．

▷口頭発表，p.156, 157

「～の原因は分かりません．この点については現在研究を進めています．」

- We are not sure why the reaction was unsuccessful. We are still checking that point.
- We are not sure why the reaction was unsuccessful. We are still looking at that issue.
- We are not sure why the reaction was unsuccessful. We are still working on that issue.

●原因を明らかにするために研究を行っているところである場合は，そのことを現在進行形で示すとよい．

▷口頭発表，p.157

「～の原因は分かりません．この点については今後の研究を予定しています．」

- We are not sure why this happens. We are planning to do further experiments on this issue.

●原因を明らかにするための研究をこれから行う予定である場合には，上記のように言う．

▷口頭発表，p.162

「この原因は分かりません．それは今回の結果が～だったからです．」

- We don't know the reason for that. Results were inconclusive.
- We don't know the reason for that. Results were difficult to interpret.
- We can't give a concrete figure. Results were mixed.

● 原因を説明できない時は，その理由を説明する．［例：inconclusive（この結果からは結論は出せない），difficult to interpret（結果の解釈が困難である），mixed（相反する結論を示す結果が混在している）］

▷口頭発表，p.157

「～の原因は分かりませんが，私達は～によるものではないかと考えています．」

- **We don't know the reason for** the difficulties in shaping alloys into new forms, **but we think that it was due to** a lack of heat control.

●はっきりとは言えないが考えられる原因はある，という場合には，上記のように「原因は分かりません」→ but →「～だと考えます（we think/guess that）」の形で説明するとよい．この方法は質疑応答の際に特に有効である．

▷口頭発表，p.160

「～の原因はおそらく～です．」

- **The reason for** the sudden increase in temperature **was probably** the increased reaction time.

●推測された原因を述べる際は，必要に応じて確信の度合いを下げる表現（probably など）を使い，「はっきりとは分からない」ことを聴衆に強調する．

▷口頭発表，p.161

「先行研究で報告されている値は約〜です.」

- In the literature, reported values are in the region of 5 to 6 percent.
- Reported values in the literature are in the region of 5 to 6 percent.

「この結果は先行研究で報告されている結果と一致しています.」

- This means that our results are in line with the literature.
- These results are pretty similar to what is in the literature.
- This result is consistent with what is in the literature.
- This means that our results are in line with reported values in the literature.

● 結果の説明においては，先行研究との比較を述べるとよい．Literature には必ず the をつけ，また不可算名詞なので s はつかないことに注意する．

▷口頭発表，p.167, 168

「一般的には／通常は～（数値など）です.」

- A typical yield is 5 to 10 percent.
- A typical duration would be 24 hours.
- Typically, cell culture time is 2 to 3 days.
- Cell culture time is typically 2 to 3 days.
- Typically, values are in the region of 5 to 10 percent.

● 学会発表，特に質疑応答においては，詳細な説明は省き，最も一般的な値のみを紹介することがある．その際は上記のような表現を用いる．

▷口頭発表，p.128, 129

「言い換えると／要するに，～です.」

- In other words, the results we got seem to have a high degree of reliability.
- To put it simply, (simple explanation).
- Basically, (simple explanation).

● 重要なポイントをより分かりやすくするためには，簡単な言葉で言い換える．

▷挨拶・口演・発表・質問・座長進行，p.33
▷口頭発表，p.125

「それについて説明するのは難しいのですが，簡単に言うと～です.」

- **It's difficult to explain. Basically,** it is a 2-step reaction with addition of a catalyst.
- **I'm not sure how to describe it. Basically,** it is a 2-step reaction with the addition of a catalyst.
- **I'm not sure how to explain it. Basically,** it is a 2-step reaction with the addition of a catalyst.

● 厳密な説明・正確な説明を行うのが難しい場合には，Basically を文頭に置いて，単純化／簡略化された説明を行うようにする.

▷口頭発表，p.163

「～であることを強調したいと思います.」
「重要なのは～ということです.」

- I'd like to stress that although the amount of nutrients in the soil increased, the yield did not decline.
- I'd like to emphasize that (important information).
- I'd like to point out that (important information).
- I'd like to draw your attention to (important information).
- The important point here is that (important information).

●注目してほしいポイントを示す際は上記のように言う.

▷挨拶・口演・発表・質問・座長進行, p.25, 42
▷口頭発表, p.148

「～だということをもう一度繰り返しておきます.」

- I'd like to go over the main points again. (review of 2~3 main points)
- I'm going to review the main points again. (review of 2~3 main points)
- So, the main points are these. (review of 2~3 main points)
- I'd (just) like to remind you of the main points so far. (review of 2~3 main points)
- This is (just) a quick reminder of the main points so far. (review of 2~3 main points)

● 重要な点を繰り返し述べることで，より分かりやすい発表になる.

▷挨拶・口演・発表・質問・座長進行，p.34
▷口頭発表，p.141

「～という専門用語は～という意味です．」

- By relapse, I mean the process where the teeth returned to their original color after treatment.
- What do I mean by relapse? Well, the term relapse refers to a change in the color of the teeth after treatment.
- Relapse, in other words, the process where the teeth go back to the original color before treatment, is a serious issue.

● 初めて出てきた専門用語は分かりやすい言葉で説明する．

▷口頭発表，p.118

「～（専門用語）は～のことと定義します．」

- **We define** relapse **as** the degree to which a tooth has reverted to its original color after treatment.
- **We define** expert assessors **as** people with over 25 years' experience of evaluation.
- Expert assessors **are defined as** people with over 25 years' experience of evaluation.
- **In this presentation, I'll use the word** degradation **to refer to** changes in color and surface roughness of the samples.
- **I'm going to use the term** degradation **to refer to** changes in color and surface roughness of the samples.

● 専門用語の説明は上記のように行うこともできる．

▷口頭発表，p.120, 121, 122

「このプロセスは～とよばれます.」

- This process is called relapse.
- This process is known as relapse.
- This process is referred to as relapse.
- This process is defined as relapse.

●1番目の例文のように called を使用する場合，as は不要（called as は誤り）なことに注意する.

▷口頭発表，p.127

「～（アクロニム）は～の略です.」

- AIST stands for Advanced Institute of Science and Technology.
- AIST is short for Advanced Institute of Science and Technology.

●アクロニム（略語）の説明には stands for または is short for のいずれかを用いる．この場合 mean は使えないことに注意する.

▷口頭発表，p.180

「～は～色で表示しています．」

- Modifications to the system **are in blue.**
- Modifications to the system **are shown in blue.**

● 文字や線の色について説明したいときは are in（＋色名）または are shown in（＋色名）と言う．

▷口頭発表，p.111

「～は～（フォント／線の種類）で示しています．」

- Values **are in** italics.
- Values **are shown in** italics.
- Values **are in** bold.
- Values **are shown in** bold.
- Values **are in** large font.
- Values **are shown in** large font.
- Values **are** underlined.

● フォント（太字，イタリックなど）の説明は，are in（＋フォントの種類）や are shown in（＋フォントの種類）と言う．

● 下線については are underlined で表す．この場合は in は入らない．

▷口頭発表，p.112

「～（記号の種類）は～を表しています.」

- The red circles **show** temperature.
- The squares **show** rate of increase.
- The dots **indicate** rate of increase.

●図表中の記号（丸，三角，矢印など）が何を示しているかは show か indicate で説明する.

▷口頭発表，p.113

「例えば～です.」

- The samples should be treated with some kind of nucleophile, **such as** alcohol or ether.
- This was calculated using variables **such as** speed, weight and mass.
- The system can be used in various ways, **such as,** medical applications.
- The system can be used in various ways, **for example/instance,** medical applications.

●具体例を示すことで聴衆が理解しやすくなる．具体例の紹介には such as，for example，for instance を用いる.

▷口頭発表，p.181

「（スライドに具体例を表示しながら）**例えばこのような例があります.**」

- **This is an example.**
- **This is an example of the reaction process.**
- **This is a typical example.**
- **Here we have a typical example.**
- **Here are some examples.**

● 口頭で例を挙げるだけではなく，具体例をスライドに表示させて説明することもできる．現在のスライドに具体例が示されている場合には，上記のように言う．

▷口頭発表，p.182

「具体例は次のスライド／セクションでお示しします.」

- I'll show you an example in the next slide.
- I'll show you some examples in the next slide.
- I'll introduce some examples of the system in the next section.
- I'll show you an example later.

● 具体例を次のスライド／セクションで示すことを予告する場合は，上記のように言う.

▷口頭発表，p.182

「この～は，例えば～に応用できます．」

- I'll just quickly mention some possible applications. The system can be used in various ways, such as, medical applications.
- I'll just quickly mention some possible applications. The system can be used in various ways, for example/instance, medical applications.

● 考えられる応用例を紹介する場合には，上記のように言う．

▷口頭発表，p.181

「はじめに～を行いました．次に～して，最後に～しました．」

- First, the samples were washed. Next, they were dried. After that they were stored. Then we calculated the difference in weight.

● 実験などの手順を説明する際は，first，next，after that，then などの順序を表す表現を活用する．

▷口頭発表，p.183

「実験に使用した装置の構成は～です.」

- This slide shows the apparatus. As you can see, it consists of (explanation).
- What is the experimental set up? It consists of (explanation).
- This apparatus consists of (explanation).

● 実験装置や実験機器については上記のように説明する.

▷挨拶・口演・発表・質問・座長進行，p.43

「これから～の動画をお見せします.」

- I'm going to show you a short video of the catalytic conversion.
- I'd like to show you a video clip of the reaction.
- I have a video clip of the reaction that I'm going to show you.
- This is a video clip of the reaction.

● 動画を使用する場合，再生前に，何についての動画なのかを簡単に説明する.

▷口頭発表，p.174

「（動画を再生しながら）**この時点では，〜です．**」

- **At this point,** the sample is stable and there is no reaction.
- **At this stage,** the sample is stable and there is no reaction.
- **Here,** the sample is stable and there is no reaction.

● 学会発表で動画を再生する場合，何らかの現象（例：化学反応）の一部始終を捉えたものであることが多い．その場合，現象の各段階について，今何が起こっているのかを口頭で説明するとよい．はじめに，動画の再生開始時点（現象が始まる前）の状態を説明する．

▷口頭発表，p.175

「(動画を再生しながら) ご覧のとおり，～が始まりました.」

- Here you can see the first stages of the reaction.
- As you can see, these are the first stages of the reaction.
- So, this is the start of the first stages of the reaction.

● 現象が始まったことを示すには上記のように言う.「ご覧のとおり，(今現象が始まりました)」は Here you can see や As you can see で表す.

▷口頭発表，p.176

「(動画を再生しながら) 続いて，～が起こります.」

- This is followed by combustion.
- And next, the sample catches on fire.
- After that, we get combustion.

● 次に起こる現象については上記のように説明する. A is followed by B は「A に続いて B が起こる」を表す.

▷口頭発表，p.176

「(動画を再生しながら) 最終的には，〜となります.」

- Finally, the sample becomes hard.
- This is the last stage of the reaction. And the sample becomes hard.
- In the end, the sample becomes hard.

● 動画の終わり（現象の終了後）の状態を説明して，動画の再生を終える.

▷口頭発表，p.176

「(動画の再生が終わった後に) この〜のポイントは何でしょうか？」

- So, what is the significance of the chemical reaction?
- We have seen various stages of the reaction. The question is, what is the significance of it?

● 動画を再生した後は，動画から読み取れるポイントを説明する．はじめに，説明を始める合図として上記のように言う.

▷口頭発表，p.177

「この動画のポイントは，～ということです．このことは～を意味します．」

- **I think we have seen that** the reaction is stable. **This means that** the process has various possible applications.
- **So, this shows that** the reaction is stable, **and** can be applied to various industrial processes.
- **This means that** the process can be used industrially for a variety of uses.

● 動画で示した内容の何が重要であったか，それが何を意味しているかについて説明する．

▷口頭発表，p.177

「すみません，訂正します．正しくは〜です．」

- Excuse me, I should have said (correct information).
- Sorry, I meant to say (correct information).
- Excuse me, that's not quite correct. I wanted to say (correct information).

「失礼しました．〜ではなく〜です．」

- Excuse me, I meant to say 150 not 250.
- I'm sorry. I should have said that temperature increased not decreased.

口頭での説明を言い間違えた場合は，謝罪→訂正の順に行う．謝罪はExcuse meかI'm sorry，訂正はI should have said（＋正しい内容）not（＋誤った内容）のように言う．

▷挨拶・口演・発表・質問・座長進行，p.46
▷口頭発表，p.179

「すみません．スライドに誤りがありました．～ではなく～です．」

- I've just seen a mistake on this slide. That should be degradable not non-degradable.
- Excuse me, that number should be 179 not 197.
- Sorry that's a mistake. It should be 179 not 197.

● スライドの内容の誤りに気づいた場合は，that should be（＋正しい内容）not（＋誤った内容）と訂正する．

▷口頭発表，p.179

「詳細については省略します.」

- I'll skip that.
- I won't go into details.
- I won't discuss this in detail.
- As time is limited, I'll skip that information.
- This slide contains a lot of information. I'll skip the detail/details.
- This slide contains a lot of data. I'll skip the detail/details.
- There is a lot of information here. I'll skip the detail/details.

説明をシンプルにしたい時や，時間が足りない時は，詳細を省いて要点のみを説明する．その際は上記のように言う．

▷挨拶・口演・発表・質問・座長進行，p.32
▷口頭発表，p.131

「詳細は省略して，重要なところだけご説明します．」

- There is a lot of information here. So, I'll skip the details and look at the main points, which are as follows: (explain the main points).
- I'll skip the details and (just) mention the important information / the key data.
- Here we have data from group 2, I won't go into details, but the main point is (explain the main point).

● 詳細を説明する時間がないときは，要点だけをかいつまんで説明する．

▷口頭発表，p.133

「時間がないので，このスライドは飛ばします．」

- I'll skip this slide.
- I'm running out of time, so I'll skip this slide.
- I only have a few minutes left, so I'll skip this slide.

● スライドを１枚丸ごと飛ばすときは上記のように言う．

▷口頭発表，p.132

「時間がありませんので，〜に移ります.」

- I'm running out of time. So, I'll move on to the discussion section.
- Since time is short, I'll go straight to the summary.

● 一部の内容を省略して次のセクションに移るときは，上記のように言う.

▷口頭発表，p.178

「申し訳ありません．1，2分オーバーしてしまいました.」

- Sorry. I think I went over by a minute or two.

● 発表時間をオーバーしてしまった場合の謝罪は上記のように行う.「(時間を）オーバーする」は go over (by＋時間）で表す.

▷口頭発表，p.178

「興味のある方は，こちらの参考文献をご参照ください.」

- If you are interested, here are the references, which give a detailed explanation of the apparatus.
- If you want to see the details, please check these references.

「こちらの URL をご参照ください.」

- I've included some relevant URLs here.
- Here are some useful URLs.
- If you are interested, please check these URLs.

● スライドに表示した参考文献・URL のリストを参照させたい時は上記のように言う.

▷口頭発表，p.164, 166

■ 発表の終わり方

「こちらが本日の発表のまとめです．」
「こちらが最後のスライドです．」

- **This is a summary.**
- **This is my last slide.**
- **This is the last slide.**
- **This is a summary of the main findings.**
- **These are the main points I covered today.**

● まとめに入る合図として，まとめスライドを示しながら上記のように言う．

▷口頭発表，p.188, 215, 225

「本日の発表のまとめをいたします.」

- I'd like to finish with a (brief) summary.
- I'd like to summarize my presentation.
- I'd like to run through the main points I made today.
- I'd like to go over the main points I covered today.
- I'd like to wrap up this presentation with a short summary.
- I want to finish by summarizing the main findings.

● まとめに入る合図として上記のように言うこともできる（前ページの例文も参照）.

▷口頭発表，p.188

「本日は〜についてお話ししました.」

- Today, I talked about water pollution in agricultural areas.
- So, we looked at water pollution in agricultural areas.
- Today, I focused on water pollution in agricultural areas.

● まとめの最初は，発表テーマを振り返る.

▷口頭発表，p.192

「この研究の目的は，〜することでした.」

- Our main objective (in this study) was to measure nitrates in rivers.
- The main aim (of this research) was to investigate nitrates in rivers.
- We wanted to analyze the levels of nitrates in rivers.

● 発表テーマの次は，研究の目的を振り返る．まとめの冒頭で研究の目的を改めて述べることで，聴衆が発表の全体像を振り返りやすくなる.

▷口頭発表，p.192, 226

「～について，特に～を中心に調べました.」

- **We looked at** the benefits of low-cost online approaches and face-to-face interventions for CVD and diabetes, **focusing on** exercise, diet, and general health.
- **We analyzed** the benefits of low-cost online approaches and face-to-face interventions for CVD and diabetes, **focusing on** exercise, diet, and general health.
- **We investigated** the benefits of low-cost online approaches and face-to-face interventions for CVD and diabetes, **focusing on** exercise, diet, and general health.

● 「特に～を中心に調べました」と言いたい時は，句動詞 focus on を用いる.

▷口頭発表，p.226

「この研究では，このような疑問に答えようとしました．」

- This is just to remind you of our research questions. What are the sources of nitrates in rivers and how can they be reduced?
- This was our research question.
- These were our research questions.
- I'd just like to remind you of our research questions, which were as follows.
- So, our research hypothesis was that sunlight is a reliable method of degrading polymers.

● まとめにおいては，リサーチクエスチョン（この研究によりどのような疑問に答えようとしたか）も振り返るとよい．

▷口頭発表，p.193

「～という手法を用いました.」

- **We used** online interviews as well as questionnaires, apps, automated reminders and community spaces.
- **We employed** online interviews as well as questionnaires, apps, automated reminders and community spaces.
- **We made use of** online interviews as well as questionnaires, apps, automated reminders and community spaces.

●方法についても簡単に再度説明する.

▷口頭発表, p.227

「こちらが本研究の主な結果です．」

- **Here are the main results. We found that** the average number of falls per patient decreased by more than 20 percent.
- **These are the main findings. We found that** (main results).
- **I'll just go over the main results. We found that** (main results).
- **These are the main results. We found that** (main results).
- **This is what we found. We found that** (main results).

● 実験結果／調査結果のうち，主なものを簡潔に紹介する．

▷口頭発表，p.194, 195, 227

「また，～ということも明らかになりました.」

- **We also found that** there are two main factors that seem to affect risk.
- **In addition, we found that** there are two main factors that seem to affect risk.
- **Additionally, we found that** there are two main factors that seem to affect risk.
- **Another thing we found was** an increase in patients' wellbeing and general happiness.

● 複数の結果を紹介する場合は，Also や In additior を用いる.

▷口頭発表，p.195, 216

これらの結果は何を意味しているのでしょうか？」

- So, what do these results mean?
- What is the significance of these findings?
- What is the meaning of these results?

● 実験結果／調査結果を紹介した後は，その結果からどのような結論を導けるかを説明する．

▷口頭発表，p.196

「これらの結果をまとめると，～です．」

- Taken together, these results tell us that action taken at grass-roots level by local staff makes a significant difference in terms of a reduction in the number of falls, and also an increase in general health and wellbeing.
- Taken as a whole, (main message).
- Overall, these data indicate that (main message).

● 「これらの結果をまとめると」と言いたい時は Taken together，Taken as a whole，Overall などと言う．

▷口頭発表，p.197

「これらの結果は，～であることを示しています.」
「これらの結果は，～であることを示しているものと思われます.」

- These results show that (conclusion).
- These results tend to show that (conclusion).
- These results appear to show that (conclusion).
- These results would appear to show that (conclusion).

● 結論の強弱は，動詞を使い分けることによって表現する．上記の例文は1番目が最も強い表現で，以下，順に弱くなる．

▷挨拶・口演・発表・質問・座長進行，p.56

「本日の発表のテイクホームメッセージは，～です．」

- **This is the take-home message.** Local initiatives involving staff are more effective than top-down directives.
- **So, the take-home message is that** the numbers of falls can be significantly reduced by involving staff in the decision-making process.
- **Here is the take-home message.** Local initiatives involving staff are more effective than top-down directives.

● 「テイクホームメッセージ」とは「家に持ち帰ってほしいメッセージ」のことで，発表を通じて聴衆に最も伝えたいメッセージのことを指す．

▷口頭発表，p.198

「本日の発表に興味をもっていただけたなら幸いです.」

- I hope that you have found this data interesting.
- I hope that this presentation will promote interest in this largely under-researched field.
- I hope that this presentation will encourage others to look at ways of creating a safe environment in care homes.

●I hope that は,「発表に興味をもっていただけたなら幸いです」「この発表が～に興味をもつきっかけになれば幸いです」のような形で発表を締めくくるのに用いる.

▷口頭発表, p.200

「本日お話ししたかったことはこれで以上です．」

- That is what I wanted to tell you today. I hope you found this data interesting.
- That is what I wanted to tell you about creating a safe environment in care homes.
- That's what I wanted to say about patient care. I hope that you found this talk interesting.
- That is what I wanted to say about patient care. I think this aspect of care necessitates further research / study.

● 発表内容が以上で終わりであることを示すには，上記のように言う．

▷口頭発表，p.200, 201

「今後の研究課題についてご紹介します．私達は今後～を行う予定です．」

- As for future work, we plan to do a study on sealants as a way of preventing tooth decay in children.
- I'd just like to mention (our) future research plans. We plan to carry out further tests on the effects of sealing teeth in young children.
- As for future work, we plan to do further experiments using lasers.
- The next step in this research is to carry out further tests on the effects of sealing teeth in young children.
- In terms of future work, we plan to do further experiments using lasers.
- I'd like to mention future directions. We are now working on ways of increasing patient access to low-cost interventions.

● まとめの最後は，今回の研究の結果を受け，今後どのような研究を行っていくつもりかを紹介する．

▷口頭発表，p.201, 202, 203, 218, 229

次の課題は〜です．」

- The next step is to refine the system with laser technology.
- The next stage is to refine the system with laser technology.
- The next stage in this research is to refine the system with laser technology.
- Our next goal is to achieve higher yields in terms of production.

今後の研究課題の紹介は，上記のように言うこともできる．

▷口頭発表，p.203

「この研究は○○基金の研究助成を受けて行いました．」

- This research was funded by the Ministry of Health, Welfare and Labor.
- For this project we are getting funding from the Dutch Program for Tissue Engineering.
- We gratefully acknowledge the financial support of Lion Corporation.
- This research/study/work was supported by a grant from the Ministry of Construction.
- I'd just like to mention that this research was supported by a grant from the Sato Foundation.
- For this research, we obtained funding from the Ministry of Education.

● 研究助成を受けて行った研究の場合は，その名称などを紹介する．利用した研究助成の種類が多い場合は次ページの例文を参照．

▷口頭発表，p.204, 219

「（スライドにリストを表示しながら）この研究はこれらの研究助成を受けて行いました．」

- **You can see our funding sources here.** (Show a list of funding sources)
- **Here are the sources of funding for this work.** (Show a list of funding sources)

利用した研究助成が複数ある場合は，スライドに研究助成のリストを提示した上で上記のように述べてもよい．この場合，リストを１つ１つ読み上げる必要はない．

▷口頭発表，p.204

「この研究にご協力いただいた皆様に感謝申し上げます．」

- I would like to acknowledge the people who worked with us on this project.
- I want to thank the people who have been involved in this work.
- I would like to thank my coworkers who have contributed to this work.
- I'd like to acknowledge my coworkers who have contributed to this work.
- I wish to thank the following people. (+ a list of names and a photo)

● 共同研究者など，研究に関わった人達への感謝の言葉を述べる．その際，共同研究者の名前のリストや写真をスライドに表示するとよい．

▷挨拶・口演・発表・質問・座長進行，p.58
▷口頭発表，p.205, 219

「ご清聴ありがとうございました.」

- Thank you.
- Thank you very much.
- Thank you for your attention.
- Thank you for your time.

「以上で発表を終わります．ご清聴ありがとうございました.」

- That's all I have to say. Thank you for your attention.
- That covers everything I want to say. Thank you.
- That concludes my presentation. Thank you.
- That covers everything I wanted to say. Thank you for your attention.

● 発表を締めくくる際は，聴衆へのお礼を述べる.

▷挨拶・口演・発表・質問・座長進行，p.57
▷口頭発表，p.206, 219, 229

『(スライドにメールアドレスを表示して) こちらが私の連絡先です．興味のある方はどうぞお気兼ねなくご連絡ください．』

- Here are my contact details. Please feel free to get in contact.
- Here are my contact details. If you are interested in this study or would like to have any more information, please get in contact.

● 自分の連絡先を紹介する際は，スライドにメールアドレスを表示した上で上記のように言う．

▷口頭発表，p.208

「何か質問はございますか？」

- I'd be happy to take any questions you might have.
- I'd be happy to answer any questions.
- Are there any questions or comments?
- I'd be pleased to answer any questions.
- If you have any questions, I'd be pleased to answer them.
- Does anyone have any questions or comments?

質問を呼びかけるのは通常は座長の役割であるが，座長がいない場合には発表者自らが質問を呼びかける．

▷挨拶・口演・発表・質問・座長進行，p.59
▷口頭発表，p.208

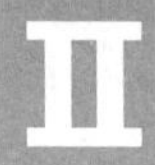

ポスター発表

「（ポスタープレビューの最後に）**ご興味のある方は，ぜひ私達のポスター発表にお越しください．**」

- **If you are interested in our study, I hope you will stop by our poster.**
- **If you are interested in this work, please visit our poster. Thank you.**

● 学会によっては，ポスターセッションに先立ち，スライドでポスター内容の概要を紹介するポスタープレビューの時間を設けていることもある．

● ポスタープレビューでは，発表内容を手短に紹介した後，ポスター発表を見に来てくれるよう上記のように呼びかけるとよい．

「こちらのポスターに興味がおありですか？」

- Hi, how are you doing?
- Hello, I'm the author of this poster. If you have any questions, I'd be pleased to answer them.

●ポスターの前を通って目が合った人には，上記のように声をかけてみるとよい．店員がよく使う Can I help you? は，ポスター会場では適当でない．

▷挨拶・口演・発表・質問・座長進行，p.122

「私のポスターにお越しいただきありがとうございます．～と申します．」

- Welcome to my poster. My name is (name).

●まずは，自分の発表に来てもらったことに歓迎の意を表する．

▷ポスター発表，p.60

「概要を説明しましょうか？」

- Can I give you a short overview of this research?
- Can I take you through this?
- Would you like me to give you a summary of the main points?

● ポスターを見に来てくれた人に対しては，概要の説明が必要か，最初に確認するとよい．

▷ポスター発表，p.63

「お聞きになりたいことはありますか？」

- Do you have any specific questions?
- Is there anything you would like to ask about?

● ポスターや抄録集に一度既に目を通している人の場合，何か質問したいことがあるかもしれない．説明を始める前に，質問がないか確認するのもよい．

▷ポスター発表，p.65

「配布資料は必要ですか？」

- Would you like a handout?
- I have a handout. Would you like one?
- Do you need a handout?

「よかったら資料をお持ち帰りください.」

- Please take a handout. This is a summary of the poster.

● 配布資料は print ではなく handout と表す.

● ポスターの前を離れる場合には Handouts: please take one と書き置くとよい.

▷挨拶・口演・発表・質問・座長進行，p.122
▷ポスター発表，p.61

「あなたは私と同じ研究分野の方ですか？」

- Are you familiar with (topic / field)?
- Are you working in this field?
- Are you working on (topic)?

● ポスターを見に来てくれた人が，自分と同じ専門分野なのかどうかによって，説明の仕方を変えるとよい．そのために，発表の前に上記のように確認する．

▷ポスター発表，p.62
▷挨拶・口演・発表・質問・座長進行，p.124

『これは〜に関する研究です．』

- This poster is about (topic).
- We did a study on (topic).
- This research concerns (topic).
- This work is concerned with (topic).
- In this study, we researched/investigated (topic).

● ポスターに立ち寄った人には，まず，何についての研究かを示す．

▷挨拶・口演・発表・質問・座長進行，p.126

『〜について研究しました．』

- We investigated/looked at (topic).
- We did some research on (topic).
- We analyzed (topic).

● 研究内容の概略は上記のように示す．

▷挨拶・口演・発表・質問・座長進行，p.128

質問がありましたらいつでも声をかけてください.」

- Please feel free to ask questions at any time.
- If you have any questions, please stop me.
- If you want to ask any questions while I'm talking, please interrupt me.
- If you want to stop me and ask a question, please do so.
- If you would like to ask a question, please interrupt me at any time.

ポスター発表においては，全部説明が終わった後に質問を受けるよりも，話の途中でもいつでも質問を受け付けるほうが好まれる．一方的にしゃべり続けるのではなく，質問をしたり話し合ったりするような「間」を与えることが大切である．そのためには，説明の冒頭で上記のように言うとよい．

▷挨拶・口演・発表・質問・座長進行，p.129
▷ポスター発表，p.64

「この研究の目的は～です.」

- The aim of this study was to investigate (objectives).
- We wanted to investigate/compare (objectives).
- In this research, we had two main goals. First, (objective). Second, (objective).

● 研究目的を明確にすることで，ポスターを見に来た人も焦点を絞りやすくなる.

▷挨拶・口演・発表・質問・座長進行，p.130

「簡単にご説明します.」

- I'd like to give a brief overview.
- I'll go over the main points of this research.
- Basically, the main findings of this research are as follows.

● 研究内容の概略を手短に示すためには，上記のように言ってから始める.

▷挨拶・口演・発表・質問・座長進行，p.131

「この図は〜を示しています.」

- Here, we have (main data from graphic).
- Here, you can see (main data from graphic).
- This figure shows (main data from graphic).
- As you can see from this chart, (main data from graphic).

ポスター内の図表について説明する際には，指や指示棒などで図表を指しながら上記のように言う.

▷挨拶・口演・発表・質問・座長進行，p.132

「詳しくはこちらの図表をご覧ください.」

- You can see the details in this figure.
- We looked at three main points: They are shown in this table.

ポスター内の図表を参照させたい時は上記のように言う.

▷ポスター発表，p.35

「ポイントを説明します．まず～です．次に～です．」

- So the main points of this section are these. Firstly, (main point). Secondly, (main point).
- The important points here are as follows. Firstly, (main point). Secondly, (main point).
- In finishing this section, I'd like to emphasize that (main point).

● 口頭での発表と同様，ポスター発表でもセクションごとにポイントを説明する．

▷挨拶・口演・発表・質問・座長進行，p.13

「ここでは詳細は省略します．」

- We're short of time, so let me skip this.
- I'll skip this.
- I won't go into details on this point.

● 詳細を省く時は上記のように言う．

▷挨拶・口演・発表・質問・座長進行，p.13

「次に～についてお話しします.」

- Next, I want to talk about (topic / data).
- In the next section, I'll show you (information).
- Now, let's take a look at the experimental apparatus.

口頭発表と同様，ポスター発表においても，次の話題に移る時はそのことを明確に示す．

▷挨拶・口演・発表・質問・座長進行，p.135

「もう一度要点を繰り返すと，～です.」

- I'd like to go over the main points again. (summary of 2~3 points).
- I'll repeat that information again. (summary of 2~3 points).
- As I already mentioned (repeat information / data).

ポスター発表においても，要点を繰り返すことは効果的である．

▷挨拶・口演・発表・質問・座長進行，p.136

「結論に移ります.」

- **I'd like to move on to the conclusion.**
- **I'd like to conclude my poster.**
- **Our main conclusions are as follows.**

●結論に移る時は，そのことを明確に示す.

▷挨拶・口演・発表・質問・座長進行，p.137

「まず（次に，最後に）～です.」

- **Firstly, we found that (main points).**
- **Secondly, our results showed (main points).**
- **Finally, this study suggests that (main points).**

●結論を述べる時は，上記のようにして要点を示す.

▷挨拶・口演・発表・質問・座長進行，p.138

「これで発表は終わりです．ありがとうございました．」

- That covers everything. I hope you found that interesting.
- That's all I have to say. Thank you.

● 口頭発表と同様，ポスター発表においても「終わり」をはっきり示す．

▷挨拶・口演・発表・質問・座長進行，p.139

「もう少し説明を加えたほうがよいでしょうか？」

- Would you like me to go over the main points again?
- Would you like any more information?
- Do you need any more information about (topic)?
- Do you want me to say a little more about (topic)?

● 発表を終える時は，説明が十分であったか確認するとよい．

▷ポスター発表，p.66

「ご理解いただけましたでしょうか？」

- Does that make sense?
- Is there anything that isn't clear?
- I hope that's clear.
- Is that clear?

● 複雑なデータなどを説明した後には，理解できたかを確認するとよい．

▷ポスター発表，p.67

「ご質問・コメントはありますか？」

- Do you have any questions?
- Do you have any comments?
- Is there anything you would like to ask about?

● 一通りポスターの説明を終えたら，質問・コメントがないかを確認する．

▷挨拶・口演・発表・質問・座長進行，p.140

「（発表の途中で聞きに来た人へ）どうぞ，今は～の話をしているところです．」

- Hi, welcome. We are talking about (topic).
- Hi, we're just talking about the results.
- Hi, I'm talking about the background.
- Hi, I'm just looking at the methods section.

● 説明や討論の途中でポスターを見に来た人に対しては，今何について話しているかを教えてあげるとよい．

▷挨拶・口演・発表・質問・座長進行，p.145
▷ポスター発表，p.100

『（これから説明する事柄についての質問を受けた場合）**それでは，次のセクションの説明に移ります．**』

- **I'd like to look at the next section. It shows details of the measurement system.**
- **Let's look at Figure 3 in the next section. It shows details of the measurement system.**
- **I want to move on to the next section. It shows details of the measurement system.**

● ポスター発表の場合，全ての説明を終える前に質問を受けることもある．これから紹介しようとしている図やデータについて質問を受けた時は，上記のように言うとよい．

▷ポスター発表，p.90

「～の話に戻りたいと思います.」

- I'd just like to go back to Table 3. As you can see, the selection process is summarized here.
- Can we go back to the methods section? As you can see, the selection process is summarized here.
- Is it okay if we have a look at Figure 2 again? As you can see, the selection process is summarized here.

● 討論の途中で当初の質問内容から話題がずれた時は，上記のように言って修正するとよい.

▷ポスター発表，p.98

「それはそうと，先ほどお話ししたとおり～です.」

- Anyway, as I was saying (summarize previous point).
- What I was saying was (summarize previous point).
- Going back to what I was saying about (topic).

● 討論のポイントがずれた時は，Anyway, as I was saying などを使って修正するとよい.

▷ポスター発表，p.99

「（論文について）後ほどメールでお送りするのでメールアドレスを教えていただけませんか？」
「（論文は）～でご覧になれます.」

- I don't have any copies with me, but I can send you the reference. Could I have your email address, please?
- My most recent paper was published in System this year. It is available online at Science Direct.

● 文献や参考文献を求められた時は，連絡先を聞いて送るように伝えるか，入手方法を教えるとよい．

▷ポスター発表，p.102

「私の発表に興味をもっていただき，どうもありがとうございました．」

- Thank you for stopping by.
- Thanks for your interest.
- It has been nice talking to you. I hope we can keep in contact.
- Thank you for your interest in my work. Let's keep in contact.

● すべてのやり取りが終わったら，上記のようにお礼を言う．

▷挨拶・口演・発表・質問・座長進行，p.146
▷ポスター発表，p.70

「コメントをありがとうございました．とても有意義な討論ができました．」

- Thank you for your comments. I enjoyed our discussion.
- Thanks a lot. I enjoyed our discussion.

● コメント・討論に対するお礼は上記のように言う．

▷挨拶・口演・発表・質問・座長進行，p.146
▷ポスター発表，p.70

「名刺をいただけますか？」「連絡先を教えていただけますか？」

- Do you have a name card with you?
- Could I have your name card, please?
- May I have your name card?
- Would it be possible to have your name card, please?
- I'd like to keep in contact. Could I have your email address, please?

● 相手の連絡先を尋ねる場合は，上記のようにすればよい．

▷ポスター発表，p.69
▷挨拶・口演・発表・質問・座長進行，p.148

「こちらが私の連絡先です．よろしければいつでもご連絡ください．」

- This is my name card. Please feel free to get in contact.
- This is my email address. I'd be pleased to hear from you.
- If you would like any more information, this is my e-mail address. It would be great to hear from you.
- If you'd like to keep in contact, please email me. Here's my name card.
- If you need more information, please get in contact. It would be great to hear from you.

● 相手と関係を築きたい時は，連絡先の記載された名刺を渡しながら，上記のように言う．

▷挨拶・口演・発表・質問・座長進行，p.147
▷ポスター発表，p.68

私の連絡先は配付資料に記載してあります.」

• My contact details are on the handout.

名刺を配る代わりに，配付資料の中に連絡先を記載するのもよい.

▷ポスター発表，p.68

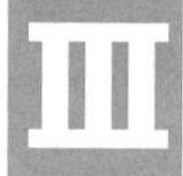

質疑応答

質問・コメント

「～番目のスライドについて質問があります．」

- I have a question about slide 7.
- My question is about slide 7.
- Could you show me slide 7, (please)?

● スライドに番号が振られている場合は，その番号を示すと，何についての質問なのかが相手に伝わりやすい．

▷口頭発表，p.84

「～についての説明がよく分かりませんでした．」

- I wasn't sure about your explanation concerning rates of recycling.

● 発表内容でよく理解できない箇所があり，もう一度説明してもらいたい場合は，上記のように言う．

▷ポスター発表，p.106

「～について質問します．～ですか？」

- I have a question about (data/figure/topic). What was the reaction temperature?
- I have a question concerning the results you showed in (figure). How do you explain the rapid increase in temperature?
- My question is about the curve shown in (figure). What does this curve represent?

● 上記のように，まず何についての質問かを明確にし，その次に質問の内容に入ると，質問内容が伝わりやすい．

▷挨拶・口演・発表・質問・座長進行，p.106

「～についてもう少し詳しく教えていただけませんか？」

- Could you tell me some more about (topic)?
- I'd like to know some more about (topic).
- Do you have any more information on (topic)?
- Could you give me some more information about medical applications?
- I am interested in sample preparation. Could you give me some more information?

● 発表を聞いてさらに詳しく知りたいと思った場合は，上記のように聞く．何について知りたいのかをはっきり示すことが重要である．

▷挨拶・口演・発表・質問・座長進行，p.108
▷ポスター発表，p.89, 96, 101

「先ほど～とおっしゃいましたが，～についてのお考えもお聞かせください.」

- You mentioned that (information / data). How do you feel about (information / topic)?
- You pointed out that (information / topic). Do you have any thoughts on (information / topic)?
- You told us that (information / topic). What are your thoughts on (information / topic)?

● 発表者に追加のコメントを求める場合，発表者が述べたことを確認してから，その上で新たなコメントを求めるという，2段階のやり方で行う.

▷挨拶・口演・発表・質問・座長進行，p.99

「～についてはどう思われますか？」

- I'm very interested in (topic). Do you have any more information on that?
- I think these problems are related. Could you comment on that, please?
- I'm wondering if this effect is caused by a rise in temperature. Do you have any ideas about that?

● 上記の例文はいずれも，1文目で何について聞きたいのかを明確にし，2文目で相手の考えを尋ねている．

▷挨拶・口演・発表・質問・座長進行，p.113

「私は～だと思うのですが，あなたはどう思われますか？」

- In my opinion, (fact/opinion). How do you feel about that?
- It seems to me that (fact/opinion). What do you think about that?
- I feel that (fact/opinion). Could you comment on that?

● How do you think about……? は誤りである．

▷挨拶・口演・発表・質問・座長進行，p.114

「～についてですが，～という解釈もできるのではないでしょうか？」

- Concerning the data in (figure), I think that this can be explained in another way. (alternative explanation).
- You showed us data from recent experiments. It seems to me there is another way of interpreting this data. (alternative explanation).
- I think there is another way of looking at this data. (alternative explanation).

● 発表で提示されたデータの解釈について，発表者と考えが異なる場合には，自分の考えを伝え，それに対する発表者の見解を聞いてみるとよい．

▷挨拶・口演・発表・質問・座長進行，p.96

『～（他の研究者／グループ）による研究結果についてはどうお考えですか？』

- **Have you considered the work done by (name / group)?**
- **How do your results compare with those of (name / group)?**
- **What do you think of the results reported by (name / group) in relation to your own results?**

● 他の研究者による研究結果についての見解を聞きたい場合は，上記のように言う．

▷挨拶・口演・発表・質問・座長進行，p.97

「～については私もそう思います．しかし～についても考慮が必要ではないでしょうか？」

- I would agree with your conclusion, but I think you need to consider (topic/information).
- I think what you are saying is correct, but in my opinion it is necessary to consider (topic/information).

● 学会発表の質問でよくあるパターンの1つは，発表者の意見に大筋で同意した上で，別の可能性を問うやり方である．

▷挨拶・口演・発表・質問・座長進行，p.98

「～との違い／関連は何ですか？」

- What are the main differences between these two techniques?
- What is the connection between the results shown in Figures 3 and 4?
- How do your results compare with those of (name of group/researcher)?

● 何かとの比較について尋ねることも，よくある質問パターンである．

▷挨拶・口演・発表・質問・座長進行，p.112

「この〜はいつごろ製品化／販売されますか？」

・How long will it be before this device is available commercially?

● 発表されている技術の製品化について尋ねたい時は available commercially という表現を使う．

▷ポスター発表，p.84

「この〜はどのような応用が考えられますか？」

・Does this membrane have any medical applications?

● 「〜分野への応用」と聞きたいときは，上記の medical の部分に分野名を入れる．

▷ポスター発表，p.85

「この研究の次の課題は何ですか？」

・What is the next step in this work?

● 今後の研究課題や研究計画を聞きたい時は，上記のように言う．

▷ポスター発表，p.93

「いえ，私がお聞きしたいことは〜についてです．〜について教えていただけませんか？」

- Actually, my question is about (topic/data). (specific question).
- I wanted to ask about (topic/data). (specific question).
- In fact, I was asking about (topic/data). Could you tell me a little more about (topic/data)?

● 発表者が質問の内容を誤解している時は，そのことを指摘して再度聞き直す．

▷挨拶・口演・発表・質問・座長進行，p.115

「大変興味深く聞かせていただきました．論文のコピーをいただけませんか？」

- I'm really interested in this study. Can I have a copy of your most recent paper?

● 発表者が学会会場に持ってきていない場合は後日メールで送ってもらうことになるので，自分の連絡先を伝えるための名刺などを用意しておくとよい．

▷ポスター発表，p.102

「先ほど～とおっしゃっていたかと思うのですが.」

- I think you mentioned that accidental falls could be reduced by staff training.
- You said the simulation took two months to set up and perform.
- So you heated the samples to 90 degrees. Is that right?

● 発表者が発言した内容について確認したい場合は，上記のように言う.

▷ポスター発表，p.86,107

「～かどうかは疑わしいと思うのですが.」

- I doubt if this method can be used with extremely thin films.

● 発表内容に対して疑義を呈したい場合は，I doubt if などと言う.

▷ポスター発表，p.108

「私は～だと考えています．」

- I have a few observations to make. Firstly, (opinion). Secondly, (opinion).
- I would like to raise a couple of points. I think that (opinion).

● 発表内容に対するコメントを述べる際の正式な（改まった）表現は上記である．

▷挨拶・口演・発表・質問・座長進行，p.94

「これはただのコメントですが，～だと思います．」

- Okay, this is just a comment. (opinion).
- Just a couple of points. (opinion).
- I'd like to make one point about (topic). (opinion).

● 発表内容に対するコメントを述べる際，少しくだけた表現を使う場合は上記のようになる．学会の雰囲気などに合わせて表現を使い分けるとよい．

▷挨拶・口演・発表・質問・座長進行，p.95

■ 質問への回答

「すみません，ご質問がよく聞こえなかったのですが.」「ご質問を繰り返していただけませんか？」

- Excuse me. I didn't catch your question.
- Could you repeat that, please?
- Would you mind repeating that, please?

● 質問が聞こえなかった時は，遠慮せずに聞き直す.

▷挨拶・口演・発表・質問・座長進行，p.66

「すみません，ご質問の意味がよく分からないのですが.」

- Excuse me. I didn't follow your question.
- Excuse me. I don't understand your question.
- Sorry. I don't follow you.

● 質問の意味が理解できない時は，分かりやすく言い換えてもらう.

▷挨拶・口演・発表・質問・座長進行，p.67

「すみません，どのスライドについてのご質問ですか？」

- Excuse me, which slide are you referring to?

● 質問者が指しているスライドを明確にしたい時は，上記のように聞く．

▷挨拶・口演・発表・質問・座長進行，p.70

「（質問中の専門用語について確認したい時）すみません，～とは何を指していますか？」

- Excuse me, what do you mean by (technical term)?

● 専門用語の意味についての確認は上記のように言う．

▷挨拶・口演・発表・質問・座長進行，p.70

「～についてのご質問ですね．」

- So this is a question about terminology.
- This is about terminology.
- So this is about terminology.

● 質問内容が長い時や複雑な時は，質問の主旨と内容を確認した上で回答するとよい．

▷ポスター発表，p.104

「～についてのご質問ということでよろしいでしょうか？」

- I guess you are asking about (topic).
- If I understand correctly, this is about (topic).
- Are you asking about (topic)?
- Is your question about (topic)?
- Are you referring to (topic)?

● 内容に確信がもてない時は，上記のように確認する．

▷挨拶・口演・発表・質問・座長進行，p.68
▷ポスター発表，p.94, 105

「それはよいご質問ですね．」

- That's a good question.
- I'm glad you asked that.
- Yes, that's an interesting point.

● 質問を歓迎することを示すには上記のように言う．

▷挨拶・口演・発表・質問・座長進行，p.141

「〜というご質問をいただきました．答えは〜です．」

- Okay, so we have a question about (topic). (repeat the question simply). (answer the question).
- This is a question concerning (topic). (repeat the question simply). (answer the question).
- Thank you. This question concerns (topic). (repeat question simply). (answer the question).

質問の意味が分かりその答えを準備できる時は，まず質問の内容を繰り返す．そうすることで，聴衆も質問の内容を再確認できる．また発表者も自分の頭のなかで答えを整理することができて，自信が芽生え冷静でいられる．

▷挨拶・口演・発表・質問・座長進行，p.73

「興味深いご意見をありがとうございます.」

- Thank you for your comment. This is an interesting point.
- You have raised a difficult point / issue.
- That's a good point.

● 答えづらい質問や意見を受けた場合は，質問へのお礼などを述べながら，回答を考えるとよい.

▷挨拶・口演・発表・質問・座長進行，p.10

「まずは最初のご質問に答えましょう.」

- Okay, I'll take your first question now.
- I'd like to answer that question now.
- Do you mind if I answer your first question now?

「では，次のご質問をどうぞ.」

- Now, I'd like to take your second question.
- What was your second question?

● 一度に複数の質問をしてこようとする人に対しては，1つずつ回答できるように質問者をコントロールする.

▷挨拶・口演・発表・質問・座長進行，p.81

「すみません，2つ目のご質問は何でしたでしょうか？」

- Excuse me, what was your second question?
- Could you remind me of your second question, please?
- Excuse me, could you repeat your second question again, please?

一度に複数の質問をされた場合，質問内容を忘れてしまうこともある．その場合は上記のように確認する．

▷挨拶・口演・発表・質問・座長進行，p.82

「最初（次の／最後の）のご質問に対する答えは～です．」

- As for your first question, (answer).
- Concerning your second question, (answer).
- About the last question, (answer).

複数の質問を受け付けた時は，上記のように1つずつ答える．

▷挨拶・口演・発表・質問・座長進行，p.83

「ご質問に対する答えは以上のとおりです.」

- **Thank you.**
- **That's all I have to say on this point.**
- **That covers everything I want to say on this point.**

● 質問に答え終わったら，はっきりそのことを示す.

▷挨拶・口演・発表・質問・座長進行，p.8

「基本的には／簡単に言うと，～です.」

- **Basically,** the main difference is the time parameters. Simulation 1 was over a period of 5 days and simulation 2 over 10 days.
- **To put it simply,** (general answer).
- **In general terms,** (general answer).

● 質問への回答をスムーズに行うためには，シンプルな説明を心がける．その際，Basically などの表現を使うとよい.

● 答えづらい質問や意見に対しては，一般論を答えてかわすとよい．この場合も，Basically や In general terms を使って，一般論であることが明確に伝わるようにする.

▷ポスター発表，p.82
▷挨拶・口演・発表・質問・座長進行，p.74, 10

「ポイントは／私が言いたかったことは〜です.」

- The point I was making was that although the thickness of the film is reduced, it is still both reliable and robust.
- My point was that although the thickness of the film is reduced, it is still both reliable and robust.
- What I wanted to say was that although the thickness of the film is reduced, it is still both reliable and robust.

● 発表内容について「○○がよく分からなかったのでもう一度説明してほしい」と言われた場合は，要点を絞って分かりやすく言い直すとよい．

▷ポスター発表，p.83

「はっきりとは答えられないのですが，おそらく～ではないかと思います.」

- I can't answer that, but I guess that (general answer).
- I'm sorry, I'm not sure, but I guess that (general answer).
- I'm afraid I can't answer that question. But I imagine that (general answer).
- We don't know the answer to that yet, but (general answer).
- Actually, I can't answer your question, but I guess that (general answer).
- That's a difficult question to answer, but in general terms (general answer).
- I'm sorry, I can't give you a precise/detailed answer, but basically (general answer).

● 正確に答えるのが難しい質問を受けた時は，その旨を伝えた上で，一般論を答える.

▷挨拶・口演・発表・質問・座長進行，p.76, 84, 143
▷ポスター発表，p.84

「すみません，それについてはまだ十分なデータがありません.」「そのご質問に対する答えは持ち合わせておりません.」

- I'm sorry, I have no data on that.
- I'm afraid I can't answer that. The data are not available yet.
- I'm sorry, but it's not possible to give you that information yet.
- Unfortunately, we have no results for that.
- That's a difficult question. I'm afraid, I can't really answer it.
- I'm afraid, we didn't look at that point/area/aspect.

● 答えられない質問を受けた時は，はっきりとその旨を伝える.

▷挨拶・口演・発表・質問・座長進行，p.77,142

「それについては本研究の範囲外なのでお答えできません．」

- Unfortunately, that isn't my field. So, I can't answer your question.
- Sorry, but that is outside the area of this study.
- Unfortunately, we didn't investigate that.

●研究範囲外の内容に関する質問を受けた時は，その旨を丁寧に伝える．

▷挨拶・口演・発表・質問・座長進行，p.78

「それについては本研究の範囲外ですが，おそらく～ではないかと思います．」

- I'm afraid we didn't look at that, but I guess that with modifications it could be used in dialysis.
- It wasn't one of the aims of this study, but I guess that (general answer).
- That's outside my field, but I guess that (general answer).

●研究範囲外の内容に関する質問を受けた時は，その旨を断った上で，一般論を答えてもよい．

▷ポスター発表，p.85

「それは複雑な問題を含んでいるので，後ほどお話ししませんか？」

- This is a complicated point. Could we talk about it later?
- This is a very complex area. Can we discuss it later?
- This is difficult to explain, but I'd be pleased to talk about it later.

●その場で回答するのが難しい時は，後で直接話す約束をすればよい．

▷挨拶・口演・発表・質問・座長進行，p.79

「申し訳ございませんが，私はそのご意見には同意できません．なぜなら～だからです．」

- I'm sorry, but I can't agree with that. (reason for disagreeing).
- Actually, I have a different opinion. (reason for disagreeing).

●質問者の意見に同意しかねる場合は，上記のように理由を説明する．

▷挨拶・口演・発表・質問・座長進行，p.103

「確かにそのように予想できます．しかし実際のデータでは～です．」

- Yes, that was what we were expecting to find, but the data shows the opposite. Actually, the yield barely increased at all.
- That interpretation is widely supported, but the data shows the opposite. Actually, the yield barely increased at all.

● 質問者の予想と実際の結果とが異なる場合には，いったん質問者の考えを肯定した上で，Actually を使って正すとよい．

▷ポスター発表，p.87

「～という点については私もそう思います．しかし～です．」

- I agree that cost is important. But there are other important factors such as reliability and durability.
- I take your point about cost. But in our study, we found there are other important factors such as reliability and durability.
- I think you are probably right about cost. But what we found was that there are other important factors such as reliability and durability.

● 質問者に対し反論したい場合には，上記のように，いったん質問者の意見に部分的に同意し，その上で自分の意見を述べるとよい．

▷挨拶・口演・発表・質問・座長進行，p.101
▷ポスター発表，p.88

「ご指摘ありがとうございます．しかし私達の見解は〜です．」

- That's a good point and something we are concerned about, but our recent results show that the system can be operated with thin films.
- I take your point about extremely thin films, but our recent results show that the system can be operated with thin films.
- I see what you mean. This is something we are concerned about, but our recent results show that the system can be operated with thin films.

● 発表内容に対する疑義を受けた時は，それを受け入れた上で見解を述べるとよい．

▷ポスター発表，p.108

「(既に説明した図表・データを再び参照する場合)～をご覧ください.」

- I'd like to go back to Figure 3. It shows that samples were prepared in a 3-step system.
- Let's go back to the data. It shows that samples were prepared in a 3-step system.
- I'd like to refer back to what I said about sample preparation. As you can see, samples were prepared in a 3-step system.

● 既に紹介した図やデータを参照させる時は，上記のように言う．その際，口頭発表の場合はそのスライドをもう一度映し，ポスター発表の場合には該当箇所を示すとよい．

▷ポスター発表，p.89

「正確な数値をお答えするのは難しいですが，お
およそ～です．」

- **It's difficult to give an exact figure, but it's in the region of 30,000 patients.**
- **It's difficult to give an exact figure, but I guess it's in the region of 30,000 patients.**
- **It's difficult to give an exact figure, but approximately 30,000 patients.**

● 学会発表の質疑応答においては，数字などを細かく正確に答えることは難しいことが多い．その場合は，上記のような表現でおおよそのところを答えるとよい．

● 「おおよそ○○」「約○○」のように概数であることを示したい場合には，in the region of を使うと便利である．

▷ポスター発表，p.92

「今後は〜について研究を行う予定です.」

- We're planning to conduct further experiments concentrating on biodegradability.
- We are going to carry out further experiments using different polymers.
- Later, we're hoping to look at biodegradability.

● 今後の研究予定について質問を受けた時は，上記のような表現で言及するとよい.

▷ポスター発表，p.93

「重要なポイントは〜です.」

- The main point is that the system is lighter and also more robust.
- The important point is that the system is lighter and also more robust.
- The main points are these: the system is lighter and also more robust.

● 質問者の理解を助けるためには，要点を述べたり，重要なポイントを強調したりするとよい.

▷ポスター発表，p.95

「先ほど述べましたとおり，～です.」

- **As I pointed out,** the government introduced new laws in 2001 and rates of recycling went up significantly.
- **As I said,** (summarize previous points).
- **As I mentioned,** (summarize previous points).

● 既に説明したことを繰り返す時は，上記のように言う.

▷ポスター発表，p.96

「～（専門用語）は，言い換えると～です.」

- The majority of it is flared, **in other words** burned off.
- The patient complained of arrhythmia, **in other words** irregular heartbeat.

● 専門用語は分かりやすい言葉で説明する．その際，in other words を使うとよい.

▷ポスター発表，p.97

「〜について少し補足します．ポイントは〜です．」

- Okay, I'd just like to add something to what I said about reliability. The point is that with minor modifications to the system, reliability is significantly increased.
- There's something else I want to say about reliability. The point is that (main point).
- Another point about reliability is that (main point).

● 質問者がデータを正しく理解していない時や同意していない時は，上記のようにポイントを絞って補足するとよい．

▷ポスター発表，p.91

「詳細は省略させていただきますが，主に～です．」

- I won't go into details, but the main application is dialysis.
- I won't discuss this in detail, but the main application is dialysis.

●時間の関係で詳細な説明ができない時は，上記のように答えるとよい．

▷ポスター発表，p.101

「いえ，私が言いたかったことは～ということです．」

- What I mean is that rates increased as a result of government regulations and also because of improvements in recycling technology.
- My point is that (main point).
- The point I'm trying to make is that (main point).

●質問者が発表内容を誤解していると思われる時には，ポイントを明確にして説明し直すとよい．

▷ポスター発表，p.106

「いえ，実際は～です.」

- Actually, we found that (correct information).
- In fact, our results show/suggest that (correct information).
- That's not quite right/correct. What we found was that (correct information).

質問者が発表内容について誤解している時は，それを正す必要がある. Actually や In fact がその合図となる.

▷挨拶・口演・発表・質問・座長進行，p.102, 144
▷ポスター発表，p.86

「例えば～です.」

- For example, using fall logbooks and fall alert stickers.
- For instance, using fall logbooks and fall alert stickers.
- Such as, using fall logbooks and fall alert stickers.

質疑応答において回答内容を補強するためには，例を挙げて説明すると効果的である.

▷ポスター発表，p.107

「このような回答でよろしいでしょうか？」
「お答えになっていますでしょうか？」

- I hope that answers your question.
- Does that answer your question?
- Have I answered your question?
- Is that okay?

● 質問に対して答えた後は，その回答でよいかどうか，質問者に確認する必要がある．そうすることで，質問者も答えが終わったことを理解できる．

▷挨拶・口演・発表・質問・座長進行，p.87
▷ポスター発表，p.103

Ⅳ 座長進行

「皆さま，おはようございます．このセッションへ，ようこそお越しくださいました．」

- Good morning ladies and gentlemen. Welcome to this session.
- Good morning. It gives me great pleasure to open today's session.
- Good morning. I'd like to open this session.

- セッション開始時の座長の挨拶は，通常，上記のように始める．
- 座長を務めるときは，セッションをできるだけ簡単にまとめることと，事前の準備を怠らないことを心がける．

▷挨拶・口演・発表・質問・座長進行，p.150

「このセッションの座長を務める～です.」

- I'd like to introduce myself. I am the chairperson for this session. My name is (name).
- Let me introduce myself. I am acting as chairperson for this session. My name is (name).
- I'm (name). I'm the chairperson for this session.

● 座長の自己紹介は不要な場合もあるが，行う場合は上記のように言う.

▷挨拶・口演・発表・質問・座長進行，p.151
▷ポスター発表，p.110

「このセッションのタイトルは～です.」

- This session is (title of the session).
- (As you can see,) the title of this session is (title of the session).

● セッションのタイトルは上記のように紹介する．読み方も含めて，事前にしっかり確認しておくようにする.

▷挨拶・口演・発表・質問・座長進行，p.152

「このセッションでは，発表〜分，質問〜分で行います．」

- Today's presentations will be 15 minutes in length. There will be 5 minutes for questions. Time will be indicated by a bell.
- I'd like to remind you of the time limits. We have 10 minutes for presentations and 3 minutes for questions.
- In this session, we have 8 posters grouped under the general topic of Regeneration. Presenters have 3 minutes presentation time. There is 2 minutes for discussion.

● 発表に先立って，発表時間と質問時間を示しておく．3番目の例文はポスター発表の場合の例で，ポスター数およびセッションのテーマも併せて紹介している．

▷挨拶・口演・発表・質問・座長進行，p.153
▷ポスター発表，p.110

「携帯電話はマナーモードにしてください.」

- Before we start, could I ask everybody to set your mobile phones to silent mode?

「携帯電話は電源を切ってください.」

- Could you please make sure you have switched off your mobile phones?
- May I ask you to switch off your mobile phones?

●携帯電話・スマートフォンについての注意も座長の仕事である. 学会のルールに合わせて上記のように行う.

▷挨拶・口演・発表・質問・座長進行, p.154

「発表者は〜先生で，タイトルは〜です.」

- I'd like to welcome (name). The title of his / her presentation is (title).
- It gives me great pleasure to welcome (name). His / her presentation is entitled (title).
- The first / next speaker is (name). The title of his / her presentation is (title).

● 発表者の名前とタイトルについては，発音も含めて事前にしっかり確認しておく.

▷挨拶・口演・発表・質問・座長進行，p.156, 157

「それでは発表をお願いします.」

- Please go ahead.
- Please start.

● 発表者の紹介を終えたら，上記のように発言して発表を始めてもらう.

▷ポスター発表，p.110

「もう時間がありません．そろそろ結論に移っていただけませんか．」

- We are running short of time. Could you conclude your presentation, please?
- I'm afraid time is almost up. Could you finish your presentation, please?
- There are only a couple of minutes left / remaining. Could you finish, please?

● 発表時間の管理は座長の重要な仕事である．残り時間が少なくなったら，上記のように言う．

▷挨拶・口演・発表・質問・座長進行，p.158

「あと～分しかありません．」

- We have 2 minutes left.

● 残り○分であることを伝えるには上記のように言う．

▷挨拶・口演・発表・質問・座長進行，p.158

「もう時間になったので，発表を打ち切ってください.」

- Time is up now.
- I'm afraid you'll have to stop there.
- I'm afraid that time is up.
- Excuse me. I'm afraid that we are out of time.
- I'm sorry, but that's all we have time for.

● 発表時間を過ぎてしまったら，上記のように言って発表を打ち切ってもらう.

▷ポスター発表，p.110
▷挨拶・口演・発表・質問・座長進行，p.159

「ご発表ありがとうございました.」

- Thank you.
- Thank you for your interesting presentation.
- Thank you very much for your informative presentation.

● 発表が終わったら，発表者へのお礼を述べる.

▷挨拶・口演・発表・質問・座長進行，p.160
▷ポスター発表，p.110, 111

「何か質問はございますか？」

- Does anyone have any questions or comments?
- The floor is now open for discussion. Are there any questions?
- We have 10 minutes for Q and A. Does anyone have any questions?

●質問を受け付けるときは上記のように言う.

▷挨拶・口演・発表・質問・座長進行，p.161
▷ポスター発表，p.111

「まだ時間がありますが，他に質問はありませんか？」

- Does anyone have any further questions?
- Are there any more questions?
- I think we have time for one last question.

●質問時間に余裕がある場合には，さらに質問を呼びかける.

▷挨拶・口演・発表・質問・座長進行，p.162

「最初の質問は～，次の質問は～，そして～の順にお願いします．」

- Okay. First question. The person at the back on the left. Next question, the person in the middle. Then, the person in the front here. Thank you.

● 質問者が多数いる場合は，上記のように取り仕切る．

▷挨拶・口演・発表・質問・座長進行，p.163

「次の質問に移ってよろしいでしょうか？」
「後ほどご討論いただくということでよろしいでしょうか？」

- Excuse me. Can we move on to the next question, please?
- Sorry, but time is limited. I'd like to move on to the next/last question.
- This is a very difficult question. Could you discuss it later?

● 発表者と質問者の意見がかみ合わないときは，次の質問に移らせてもらう．

▷挨拶・口演・発表・質問・座長進行，p.164

「質問の内容は～についてです．」

・The question is (repeat question).

「申し訳ございませんが，質問を繰り返していただけませんか？」

・Excuse me. Could you repeat your question, please?

「次の質問に移ってもよいですか？」

・Could we move on to the next question, please?

● 発表者が質問の内容を理解できていない時や発表者が答えられない時は，上記のように座長が助け船を出すとよい．

▷挨拶・口演・発表・質問・座長進行，p.165

「すみません，もう少し大きな声で話していただけますか.」

- **Excuse me. Could you speak more loudly, please?**
- **Just a moment please. Someone will bring a microphone.**

● 質問者の声が小さい場合に注意するのも座長の仕事である．2番目の例文のように，スタッフにマイクを持って行ってもらうのもよい．

▷挨拶・口演・発表・質問・座長進行，p.166

「申し訳ございませんが，質問を短くまとめていただけませんか.」

- **Excuse me, time is limited. Could you state your question briefly, please?**
- **Excuse me, time is limited. Could you be more to the point, please?**

● 質問者に対し，質問を短くしてほしい時は，上記のように言う．

▷挨拶・口演・発表・質問・座長進行，p.167

「申し訳ございませんが，答えを短くまとめていただけませんか.」

- I'm afraid that time is limited. Could you give a short answer, please?
- Excuse me. We are running short of time. Could you finish your answer, please?

● 発表者に対し，答えを短くしてほしい時は，上記のように言う.

▷挨拶・口演・発表・質問・座長進行，p.168

「申し訳ございませんが，時間がありませんので質問は 1 つだけにさせていただきます.」

- I'm afraid time is very limited. We have time for one quick question.

「申し訳ございませんが，時間がありませんので次の演題に移らせていただきます.」

- I'm afraid there is no time for any questions. I'd like to move on to the next presentation.

● 質問の時間がとれないときは，上記のように取り仕切る.

▷挨拶・口演・発表・質問・座長進行，p.169

「私から１点質問させていただきます．～でしょうか？」

- I wonder if I could ask a question. Can this method be applied to (other products)?
- Excuse me. May I ask a question? What are the main applications of this technique?
- I have a question. When will this product be available?
- I have one question. When will this product be available?
- I'd like to check one point. Was the experimental setup the same in both experiments?

● 質問が少なかったり，何も質問がない時は，上記のように座長自ら質問する．

▷挨拶・口演・発表・質問・座長進行，p.170
▷ポスター発表，p.111

「他に質問はないようですね.」

- Okay, so there aren't any questions.
- There don't appear to be any questions.
- I don't think there are any more questions.

● 一通り質疑応答が終わったら，他に質問がないことを確認する.

▷ポスター発表，p.111

「質問がないようですので，この発表は終わりにします.」

- I don't think there are any more questions. Thank you very much.
- Okay, there don't appear to be any more questions. Thank you very much.

● 質問がない時は，上記のようにして発表を終わらせる.

▷挨拶・口演・発表・質問・座長進行，p.171

「それでは次の演題に移ります．発表者は〜，タイトルは〜です．」

- The next presentation will be made by (name). The title is (title). (name). Thank you.
- The next presenter is (name). His/Her presentation is entitled (title). (name). Thank you.

次の発表に移る時は上記のように言う．

▷挨拶・口演・発表・質問・座長進行，p.172

「それでは次のポスターに移ります．発表者は〜，タイトルは〜です．」

- That's all we have time for. I'd like to move on to the next poster. The next presenter is Dr. Keiko Suzuki. Would you start, please?
- Let's move on to the next poster. Dr. Watanabe, please go ahead.
- I'd like to move on to the next poster.

ポスター発表の場合は，次の発表に移る時は上記のように言う．

▷ポスター発表，p.111

「次の演題は急遽中止になりました．」

- **The next presentation has been cancelled. (announce next presentation).**

● 演題の取り下げや発表者の欠席などがあった場合は，上記のようにアナウンスし，次の演題へと移る

▷挨拶・口演・発表・質問・座長進行，p.17

「これでこのセッションを終わりにします．どうもありがとうございました．」

- **I'd like to close this session by thanking all the presenters/speakers for their contributions.**
- **This session is now closed. Thank you very much.**
- **That's the end of this session. I'd like to thank the presenters and everyone who attended. It has been a very interesting session. Thank you very much.**

● セッションを終わらせるときは，発表者へのお礼を含めて上記のように言う．

▷挨拶・口演・発表・質問・座長進行，p.17
▷ポスター発表，p.11

「いくつかお知らせがございます．まずは明日の時間についてです．明日は 9：00 より始まります．総会は 11：00 よりメインホールで行います．今夜はこのあと 7：30 より，メインホールで懇親会を行います．」

- I have several announcements that I would like to make. First, about the starting time for tomorrow. The first session will begin at 9:00 am. Second, the plenary scheduled for 11:00 am will take place in the main hall. Also, I'd like to remind you that the banquet starts in the main hall at 7:30 this evening.

● セッションの終わりに，座長として学会の連絡事項を述べることもある．その場合は上記のように案内する．

▷挨拶・口演・発表・質問・座長進行，p.175

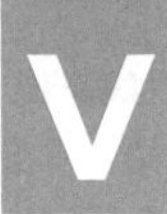

授賞式・懇親会

■ 授賞式（審査結果発表・受賞スピーチ）

「それではご注目ください.」

- May I have your attention, please?

● 審査結果発表を始めるにあたり，はじめに聴衆の興味を引きつけるために上記のように言う.

▷ポスター発表，p.115

「本学会では，毎年最も優れたポスター発表にポスター賞を授与しています.」

- Each year at this conference, there is an award for the best poster presentation.

● 審査結果発表の前に，賞の概要を簡単に説明する.

▷ポスター発表，p.115

「審査員は～名で，評価基準は以下のとおりです．」

・There are ten judges and the criteria are as follows: the poster can be understood by non-specialists, has good layout, balance between text and visuals, logical presentation, and clear and concise supporting explanation.

● 審査員の人数や評価基準など，賞の審査に関する情報を簡単に説明する．

▷ポスター発表，p.115

「今年は全部で～つのポスター発表がありました．」

・This year, there were 279 posters.

● 評価対象の総数を読み上げる．

▷ポスター発表，p.115

「全体的にとてもレベルが高く，ポスター賞の審査は非常に難航しました．」

・Standards have been very high and the judges have had a difficult time selecting the best poster.

●このように述べることで，発表者全員の努力を称える．

▷ポスター発表，p.115

「受賞者の方をご紹介します．今年のポスター賞は，～さんの～についてのポスターです．～さん，ご登壇ください．」

・I would now like to announce the winner. This year the award goes to Dr. Jun Tanaka for his poster on cell signaling. Dr. Tanaka, would you come forward, please?

●受賞者の名前と発表内容を紹介した後，受賞者に登壇を促す．

▷ポスター発表，p.115

「第〜回〜学会ポスター賞を贈ります．おめでとうございます．」

• It gives me great pleasure to present this award to Dr. Jun Tanaka at this the 15th annual JASMEE conference. Congratulations.

● 壇上における表彰時には上記のように言う．

▷ポスター発表，p.115

「受賞スピーチをお願いします．」

• Could you say a few words, please?

● 受賞者にスピーチを依頼する．

▷ポスター発表，p.115

「このような栄誉ある賞をいただき，大変光栄に存じます.」

- It is a great honor to receive this award.

● 受賞スピーチでは上記のように改まった表現を用いるのがよい.

▷ポスター発表，p.117

「この研究は多くの皆さんのご協力に支えていただきました.」

- I would like to stress that the work presented in the poster is the result of contributions by a number of people.

「共同研究者の皆さんのご協力に深く感謝申し上げます.」

- I would like to take this opportunity to thank my colleagues for their support.

● 受賞スピーチでは，共同研究者などお世話になった関係者への謝辞も述べるとよい.

▷ポスター発表，p.117

懇親会の司会

「皆さん，こんばんは．懇親会にご出席いただき誠にありがとうございます．司会の～と申します．」

- Good evening, ladies and gentlemen. Welcome to this banquet. My name is (name) and I am a member of the organizing committee.

● 懇親会の最初の挨拶は手短に済ませる.

▷挨拶・口演・発表・質問・座長進行，p.178

「今夜はゆっくり楽しんでいただきたいと思います．」

- I hope that you have had a great conference so far. I'm very pleased to see so many people here tonight.

● 上記のような，一般的な挨拶もつけ加える.

▷挨拶・口演・発表・質問・座長進行，p.179

「基調講演をしていただきました〜大学の〜先生をご紹介いたします.」

- There are a number of people I would like to introduce. First, our keynote speaker, (name), from (university name).

● 重要な方を紹介する時は，上記のように言う.

▷挨拶・口演・発表・質問・座長進行，p.180

「〜先生，どうぞ前へいらしてご挨拶をお願いできますか.」

- (name), would you be kind enough to come to the front and say a few words?
- I'd like to ask (name) to come to the front and say a few words.

● 来賓に挨拶をお願いしたい時は，上記のように言う.

▷挨拶・口演・発表・質問・座長進行，p.181

「〜先生，ありがとうございました.」

- Thank you very much, (name).

● 来賓の挨拶が終わったらお礼を述べる.

▷挨拶・口演・発表・質問・座長進行，p.182

「～（会議の運営に関わった人）にお礼申し上げます.」

- I would like to thank everyone who helped us to organize this conference.
- I would like to thank our sponsors, (name of sponsors). (Also), I would like to say how grateful I am to our keynote speakers.

● 運営に携わっている人への謝辞は，上記のように言う.

▷挨拶・口演・発表・質問・座長進行，p.183

「それでは，前途を祝して乾杯を行いたいと思います．」

- I would like to propose a toast. To the continued success and development of our society, and to its members. Cheers. Or, as we say in Japanese, *kanpai*.

● 乾杯の挨拶は，上記のように行う．「乾杯の音頭をとる」は propose a toast で表す．

▷挨拶・口演・発表・質問・座長進行，p.184

「それでは，～先生に乾杯のご発声を頂戴いたしたいと思います．」

- I would like to call on (name) to propose a toast. (name). Thank you.
- I would like to ask (name) to propose a toast. (name). Thank you.

● 誰かに乾杯の発声を頼む時は，上記のように言う．

▷挨拶・口演・発表・質問・座長進行，p.185

「お知らせがございます．明日のセッションは
9：00 の開始となります．」

• I'd like to make some announcements. Can I remind you that the first session will start from 9:00 am tomorrow?

「お知らせがございます．この会場からホテルまでのシャトルバスをご用意しております．」

• Also, I'd like to inform you that a shuttle bus will operate from the conference center to the hotel directly after this banquet finishes.

● 懇親会の司会では連絡事項に関するアナウンスも必要である．

▷挨拶・口演・発表・質問・座長進行，p.186

「それではこれで懇親会をお開きにしたいと思います．どうもありがとうございました．おやすみなさい．」

・I would now like to close this banquet. Thank you very much for attending. Good night.

・I'm afraid, we have to close this banquet now. I hope you have had a good time. Thank you for coming. Good night.

● お開きの挨拶は上記のように行う．

▷挨拶・口演・発表・質問・座長進行，p.187

【著者略歴】

C.S. Langham

1976 年　ハダースフィールド大学卒業
1982 年　ケント大学大学院修了
2000 年　日本大学歯学部教授（英語）
2020 年　日本大学特任教授

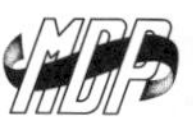

国際学会 English　ポケット版
ISBN978-4-263-43367-6

2022年 7月20日　第1版第1刷発行

著　者　C.S. Langhar
発行者　白　石　泰

発行所　医歯薬出版株式会
〒113-8612　東京都文京区本駒込1－7－
TEL. (03)5395－7638(編集)・7630(販売
FAX. (03)5395－7639(編集)・7633(販売
https://www. ishiyaku. co. jp
郵便振替番号 00190－5－138

印刷・あづま堂印刷／製本・愛千製本